ACCLAIM FOR *RYAN FARRELL'S*

GOD MADE ME SPECIAL

"Ryan is a young active member of St. Mary's Catholic Church. He has written a book about living with Tourette syndrome which is a story that needs to be told. The fact that Ryan writes for other young people makes the book interesting, but the fact that his writing increases sensitivity to children with special challenges makes the book important. Ryan's book will be a valuable service to children and to all of us who seek a better understanding of one another."

Father Todd M. Riebe,
Richmond Catholic Community,
Richmond, IN

....

"When Ryan shared his text with me earlier this year, I was surprised. My reaction was not because he had written a book, but because of the quality of his work. He truly went out on a limb to share his personal self with the reader. His story is nothing less than inspirational."

Mrs. Kathyrn Schlichte, Principal,
Seton Catholic School, Richmond, IN

"Ryan allowed me to review the book which he has written. In truth, I was completely astounded. I have never had the opportunity of being able to learn what an 11 year old feels when he/she has a disorder such as Tourette. In spite of my having been involved with almost 1,000 children and adolescents with this disorder, I have never before had as clear an understanding of the impact that this disorder has on a person. I found this book to be a very inspiring story and I feel that it would be of great help to many other families with a similar situation."
Dr. Gerald Erenberg,
Pediatric & Adolescent Neurology,
Cleveland Clinic Children's Hospital.

God Made Me Special

God Made Me Special !!!!

Tourette Syndrome

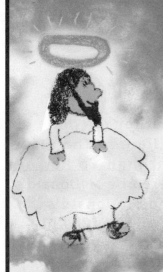

My Personal Story
By Ryan C. Farrell

Children
Writing for
Children

CWC Mission Statement

Children Writing For Children is dedicated to supporting the value of children through educational programs, scholarships, grants and by providing real publishing opportunities for their work.

CWC On The Author

Ryan Farrell is also the author of two award winning essays. He won 2nd place in the 1996 Breaking Through To Be Your Best Essay Contest sponsored by McDonald's nationwide. Ryan received McDonald's coupons and a Sports Illustrated for Kids subscription. In 1995 the Wayne County Mental Health Association sponsored an Essay Contest for approximately 850 entrants, ages 5th to 8th grade. Ryan won 1st place and received free McDonald's food for one year.

CWC publishes works written by children on specific subjects which explore the causes and consequences of today's social problems.

CWC is proud to have such a story in Ryan's God Made Me Special.

Dedication

To Nick: For being the best brother that I could ever have hoped for. Through thick and thin we have stuck together no matter what. Although we may get into fights at times, I hope you know that I will always love you. I want to thank you for defending me when others were cruel to me and for being my best friend.

To Mom: For being the most understanding and special person in my life. From the moment you had me up until now, never once have you stopped loving me. I want you to know that I love you that much and more because you have always been so patient with me and helped me when I was sad. You are truly a saint in my eyes.

Special Thanks

Dr. Gerald Erenberg of the Cleveland Clinic
The Cleveland Clinic Foundation
Bank One
Dr. Linda Ronald and Fr. Todd Riebe
Grandma and Grandpa Coffee
Grandma and Grandpa Farrell
My Mom, Dad and Nick
My family, close friends and Scout Leaders
Mrs. Hollingsworth and Mrs. Badgley
Miss Pace and Mr. William E. Williams
God

Ryan

Children Writing For Children extends its heartfelt appreciation and gratitude to the following for their time, energy and support: Prepress Advisor & Graphics Editor, Alice Byrne; Editors, Leah Hackleman, Ph.D., Elizabeth Young & Sarah Ward; The Farrell Family, Bank One; Terry Freeman & Lory Jenkins.

A special thanks to Jack Kreber and Kreber Graphics of Columbus, Ohio for generously contributing to the support of Ryan's book by donating prepress materials, use of equipment, and professional expertise.

FIRST EDITION   ISBN: 1-884825-22-2

FOREWORD

I am thankful for the opportunity to have written the foreword for this exciting book. I have been privileged to see the many advances that have been made in the field of Tourette syndrome during the time I have been involved with this neurological disorder.

These advances have been on the human side as well as the scientific. I believe that Tourette syndrome was the first medical disorder which was once considered rare, but which is now recognized as being common.

Through the efforts of support groups which arose to help spread knowledge about Tourette syndrome, the efforts of persons with Tourette syndrome and their families, and the Tourette Syndrome Association, the word has spread among communities that there are persons who have a unique neurological disorder. This has encouraged persons with Tourette syndrome to speak out and demand that they be recognized as individuals with the same strengths and weaknesses as the rest of us. There has also been a slow but steady increase in the number of publications written by persons with Tourette syndrome to describe what their life has been like. These have mostly been written from the perspective of those who are now adults. In the past, the experience of being a child with Tourette syndrome has been chronicled in several books by parents of such children, but Ryan's contribution is exciting and unique because it presents to the world what it is like to be a child with Tourette syndrome.

Although I have met more than a thousand children with Tourette syndrome, I never cease to be amazed at the resilience and resourcefulness they possess. Reading Ryan's book has again emphasized the need for professionals to be humble in the face of their patients who endure much more that we can imagine but do so with grace and resourcefulness.

I am proud to have been associated with Ryan and his family, and I am certain that he will be successful throughout his life.

Gerald Erenberg, M.D.
Pediatric Neurologist
Cleveland Clinic

PREFACE

I am very pleased to be asked to write a few words about Ryan Farrell's book on Tourette syndrome. Ryan has been a pleasure to work with and has taught me a great deal. Not only is he a fountain of information about hunting and golf, subjects which I was not very familiar with, but he has shown me new ways to think about this very difficult disorder.

Ryan continues to struggle with being teased and frustrated, but each time we talk, I hear plans about the future and see Ryan's efforts to find positive aspects of Tourette. This book will never really have an end... because Ryan will be crafting new chapters with each new challenge he tackles. My hope is that it confirms the experiences of all who read it and encourages you to engage your own "life story," whether you have Tourette, or care about someone who does, because you're special too!

Linda Ronald, Ph.D.
Psychologist
Richmond, IN

chapter one

Tourette Syndrome - My Personal Story

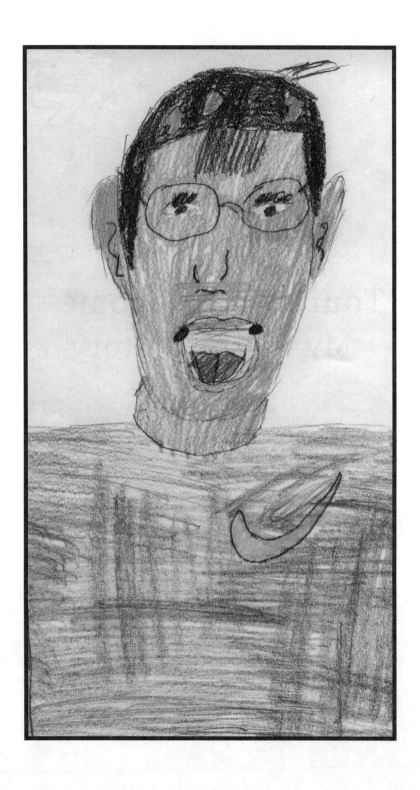

"What on earth is Tourette syndrome," you ask? That's a tough one! Tourette is a neurological (brain) disorder characterized by sudden jerks or movements, vocal and motor tics, Obsessive Compulsive Disorder, and a Conduct Disorder. Many Tourette patients also have ADHD (Attention Deficit Hyperactive Disorder), echolalia (repeating things that other people say), and in some severe cases, coprolalia (shouting of bad words involuntarily). Well, guess what? I have all of the above except coprolalia (shouting bad words).

Hi, I'm Ryan. I'm twelve years old and I'm in the sixth grade. I would like to tell you about my Tourette syndrome.

First of all, I have tics, which are facial movements and not the ones found on animals. I stretch my mouth open all the way until it hurts and I stick out my tongue at the same time. Sometimes I use my fingers to help do the stretching. This causes sores to form on the sides of my mouth. They often become infected, so I have to keep lip ointment on the sores at all times. I also widen my eyes, twitch my nose and rub my nose excessively with my thumb and index finger. I have one vocal tic and it is sniffing my nose. I sound like I have a cold all of the time. Why I do these things is hard to explain. I get a tingly feeling that starts in my mouth, so I stretch it wide, than the feeling moves into my head, then my scalp and it comes out with my hair when I pull it out. This happens when I'm overwhelmed with school work, when I'm around a lot of people or sometimes when I'm bored.

I also have obsessive compulsive behaviors which are even more difficult to deal with. I pull out the hair on my head. Sometimes I pull my hair by a single hair, sometimes in clumps. I don't just rip them out and throw them on the ground, I look at them first. Again, it's the tingle inside me that makes me do this and if I try to stop pulling my hair I become completely miserable. Sometimes I obsess about a word or a number

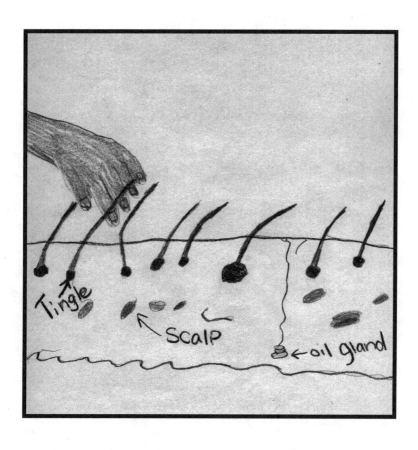

until it drives me nuts and I will pull a hair out of my head to get rid of the word or number. Pulling my hair can be quite painful, but it's worse on me if I do not pull the hair out.

Not all of my obsessions are painful to me. Some make me happy. For example, I love to hunt and I'm a great hunter. I hunt whenever I can. I watch videos on hunting with a pointer dog, read books and magazines on hunting, write reports in school on hunting, and talk nonstop about hunting. My latest hunting obsession is squirrels.

In the spring and summer I'm just as obsessed about golf. I do everything from taking lessons to playing daily. I also have an obsession of the Civil War. I have read almost every Civil War book there is. I go on trips to visit battle grounds and burial sites of the Civil War. I also am a drummer boy for an Indiana Reenactment Unit. I have marched in two parades with my Unit already and I have others coming up. Basically, I give 200% to my obsessions, whatever they are. I add to them all of the time.

Another part of my Tourette is called "Conduct Disorder." This means I can't control my temper when I want to. I throw fits when I don't get my way about something. I get miserable when I do this because I don't like acting this way. I try to stop, but that only makes it worse and that's when I moan and whine. My parents tell me to stop, but I can't. I also have ADHD. These letters stand for "Attention Deficit Hyperactive Disorder." It means I can't pay attention for long periods of time. I am constantly fidgeting or moving around and I get distracted very easily. It makes school work next to impossible. ADHD also makes me hard to get along with because I'm so impulsive. I do and say whatever comes to my mind and sometimes that gets me into a lot of trouble.

"Echolalia" is the other part of Tourette that I deal with. Often when people say things that catch my attention, I feel the need to repeat exactly what they said. I used to repeat the words in a whisper to myself, but now I have switched to repeating the words in my head so that no one can hear them. I changed because I was afraid of being

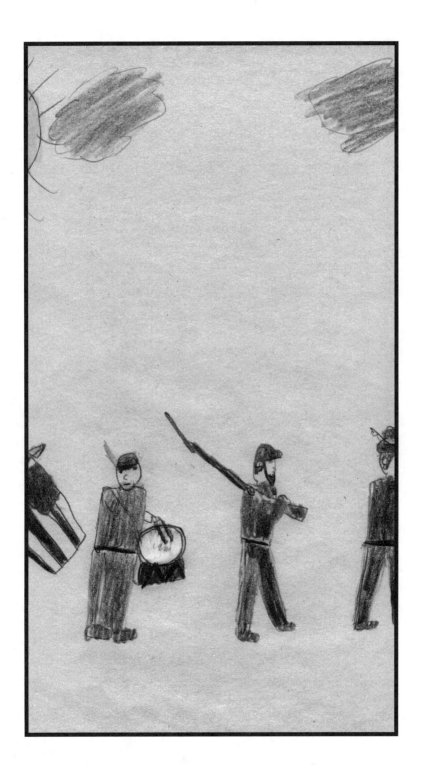

teased or questioned. Echolalia also bothers me when I'm reading. My eyes keep reading the sentence over and over again. I feel confused and stupid when this happens.

I'll bet you'd like to know how I got Tourette? It was genetically passed to me through my parents. It is such a complex disease that doctors cannot pinpoint what is responsible. They are always doing research to try to isolate specific genes, which may someday lead to a cure. I also believe God gave me Tourette to help make me truly special when I grow up. There aren't many people that are capable of dealing with my problem and that's why I think God made me special.

I will endure Tourette for the rest of my life, but it may get better with time. It also could get worse. I do not want sympathy. I just want to tell my story and help others who have Tourette or think they might have Tourette. This book is for them.

••••••••••••••••••••••••••

chapter two

The Early Years

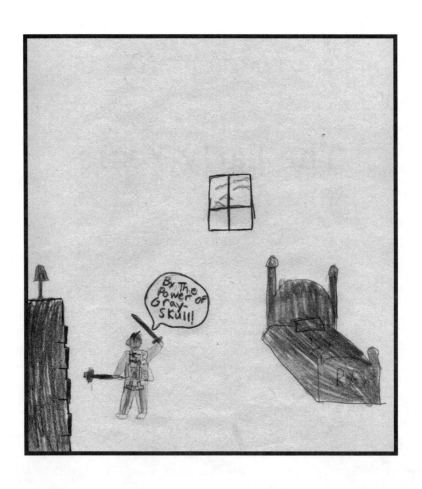

I can remember as far back as five years of age. I wasn't a happy child because I was always in trouble with my parents for being bad. I can remember lying to get out of trouble. One story comes to mind when I was five years old and in Kindergarten.

My school was having a pizza sale. Each day when the teacher asked how many pizzas we had sold, I said numbers like 15 one day, 25 another day and so on. My teacher then asked my mother if I had really sold all of those pizzas. Of course, when my mom said "No, I hadn't sold that many pizzas," I was caught. My punishment was an early Christmas present that my grandma gave me was held back until Christmas. That was hard on me because I do not like to wait for anything (except for shots)!

I was always in trouble during the holidays. As I just said, my Tourette makes it hard for me to wait for anything. Waiting for Christmas was torture. I couldn't sleep or concentrate in school. The same was true for spring and summer vacation or my birthday. I acted up and did poorly in school, but I couldn't help myself.

I can also remember really being into the "HeMan" characters at age five. The "HeMan" toys were probably part of my obsessive compulsive behavior. I carried around the tiger named "Battle Cat" everywhere I went. I didn't like to get him wet, so I set him outside the tub while I took a bath. I also slept with "Battle Cat" by my side and a "HeMan" sword down the back of my pajamas. I did this because I always liked being exactly like the characters I played with.

I can remember dressing up like people I looked up to, such as Mr. Klem, the school principal at the time, my grandfather and my dad. I also dressed up like Captain Hook and "Magnum, P.I." (Tom Selleck). I would use stuff I found laying around in my closet to make the costumes I wore.

Another memory is smelling things. Whenever I picked up food, a toy or a book, I smelled them first. I can remember having to do this in order to feel right, but I can't explain why.

School was rough for me. It seems I was always in trouble with the teachers, too! In the first and second grades I was labeled the "class clown" because I often would talk out of turn and interrupt the teacher. I also back-talked to them when they corrected me. I did this because I was angry about being corrected. I didn't then and still do not like to be told what to do. I understand that I need to be corrected, but I still do not like it when it happens.

I went to a private school until the third grade and then my parents had me tested for ADHD because I had trouble paying attention, doing my work and behaving. I can remember being pulled out of my third grade class by the social worker and she announced in front of my whole class that I was being tested for ADHD. I was very embarrassed and real mad at this woman. We found out then that I did have ADHD. My family and I then went into private counseling to try and help me. The counselor aggravated me, because she blamed me for making my family miserable, but I guess she helped my parents because she made suggestions that would help with my behavior problem.

My parents decided that I should repeat the third grade because I was young and needed a year to grow. My younger brother, Nicholas, and I were switched to a public school that next school year. I still talked out of turn, but the teacher was more patient with me.

I didn't have many friends there, but I liked the friends I met there really well. My grades improved and I was more relaxed. I didn't get to stay at my new school for very long because my dad got a promotion and we moved to a new city at the end of the third grade.

This new school is the one I'm in now and it is even better than my last school. This one is another private school. The kids in my fourth grade class were much nicer and the classes were smaller. My teacher, Mrs. King,

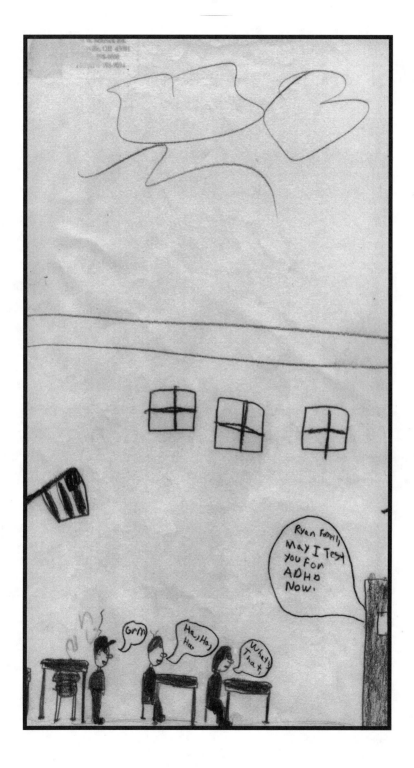

was loving and made me feel pretty good about myself.

About half the way through the fourth grade, my mom noticed that I was stretching my mouth and sticking out my tongue at the same time. I didn't know that I was doing this. I also had a bald spot about the size of a quarter on the back of my head. I didn't remember pulling my hair out at all. My parents took me to the barber to a get a buzz. They thought that this would make me stop pulling my hair our. It didn't. My spot just grew bigger and bigger. They knew something else had to be wrong with me.

•••••••••••••••••••••••••

chapter three

The Diagnosis

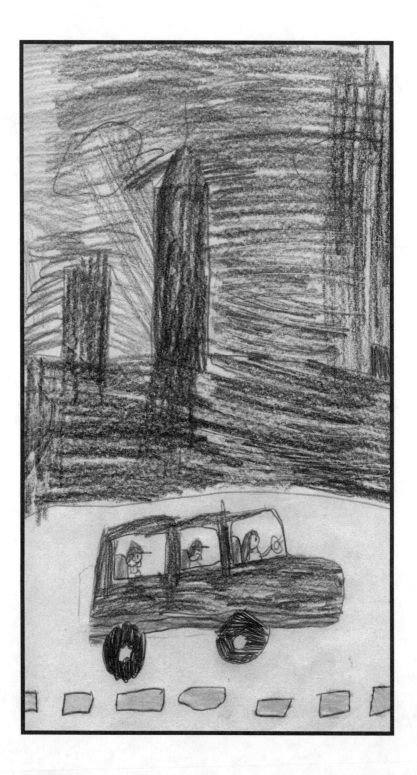

My mother was talking with my best friend's mother, Mrs. Badgley, about all of the strange things I had been doing. Mrs. Badgley told my mom about a wonderful doctor friend of hers who counsels children. She told my mom that she would ask Dr. Ronald (her friend) if she knew what was wrong with me. Well, Dr. Ronald called my mom. She told my mom immediately that it sounded like I had Tourette syndrome. She suggested that we call the Cleveland Clinic Foundation in Cleveland, Ohio. They specialize in pediatric neurological disorders (children's brain disorders).

My mom called the Cleveland Clinic and scheduled an appointment for me to get diagnosed. Mrs. Badgley and her son Kyle (my best friend) also scheduled an appointment at the Cleveland Clinic. Kyle has Dyslexia and he was going to be tested for Attention Deficit Hyperactive Disorder.

The four of us took off the last day of school and drove for three and one-half hours of the four hour trip. We stayed in a hotel the night before our appointments. We got to have a pizza party in our room and swim in the hotel pool. Our moms kept throwing change into the pool. Kyle and I dove for the change. We split the money and played four video games with it. We had a lot of fun together. I'm glad I have the mom I have. She really loves me.

The next morning Kyle and I went to our appointments. I was extremely nervous because I was afraid that if I did have Tourette, how was I going to explain it to all of my friends and classmates? I was also afraid of meeting this new doctor because I didn't know what he was going to do to me.

My doctor's name is Gerald Erenberg. He is a pediatric neurologist. When I met Dr. Erenberg, he asked me what my name was. He asked me how I was doing and basically made me feel comfortable. Dr. Erenberg then put me through some simple neurological tests. He made me hop on one foot, then the other. He made me walk in a straight line, one

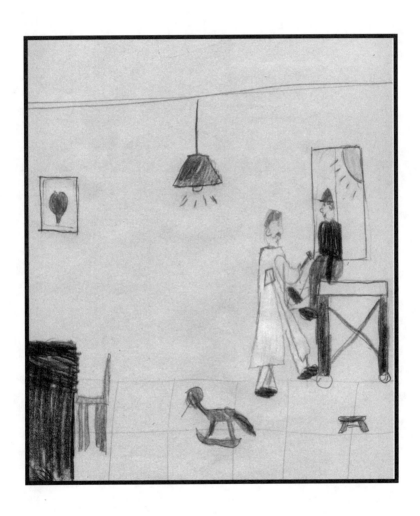

foot in front of the other. He also checked my reflexes and did other tests of my eyes. Dr. Erenberg explained to my mom and me that the real testing for Tourette comes from my personal history.

He began asking questions to my mother about being pregnant with me and my birth. He also asked questions about my childhood and my school records. I didn't really pay much attention to the two of them talking. I just sat there until Dr. Erenberg wanted to talk to me. I can remember sitting behind Dr. Erenberg and doing my tics so that he couldn't see me. I was embarrassed for him to see me. When it was my turn to talk, Dr. Erenberg asked me how I was treated in school. I told him that some of the kids in my school had been making fun of my bald spot and the faces that I make. Dr. Erenberg then explained to me that I have Tourette syndrome because of the things that my mom had just told him.

He asked me what I wanted him to do for me. I told Dr. Erenberg that I wanted him to take my tics away so that kids would quit making fun of me. He said he would try to do that, but it would mean that I had to take medication. I said that was just fine as long as it would work. I'm sure that Dr. Erenberg thinks I'm special too because he gave me his business card and told me to call him whenever I need him. I haven't had to call him yet, but it feels good knowing that I can.

When we left Dr. Erenberg's office, my mom seemed really excited because she now knew the reason why I was doing these strange things. I was happy too because now I knew that I wasn't going crazy. I really felt like I was with people teasing me and pointing out my behaviors and bald spots. Since the diagnosis, I know the things that I do are O.K. I then asked my mother if she would try and have a little more patience with me from then on. My mom had tears in her eyes and she said, "sure."

Oh, by the way, Kyle was diagnosed with ADHD and he is taking medication to help him concentrate in school. He is doing just fine.

························

chapter four

My Treatment

We found out that I have Tourette syndrome—that was the easy part. Fixing my Tourette is the tough part. My treatment involves taking medication, visits to my therapist, Dr. Ronald, and meeting with other friends that have Tourette syndrome. I'd like to tell you a little bit about these three things.

First of all, Dr. Erenberg, my neurologist, put me on a medicine called "Chlondine." This medicine has been known to treat all four of the areas of my Tourette. If you can't remember what they are, I'll tell you. Motor and Vocal Tics, Obsessive Compulsive Disorder, ADHD and Conduct Disorder. I started taking one half of a pill once a day for a week. I then had to add another half of a pill for a week. The third week I added another half of a pill. My parents had to call Dr. Erenberg at the end of three weeks to let him know if the medicine was working and if it had any side effects. It did. I was getting dizzy and really tired.

My body adjusted to the medicine after a few more weeks. The medicine did help with my behavior and ADHD. I know my parents were proud of that. It didn't do anything for my tics or for my obsessive compulsive behavior though. Since it was summer and I wasn't under the stress of school, it didn't matter to us that I was still doing my tics and pulling out my hair. That only matters during the school year when kids make fun of me.

In October, 1994 (four months after my first visit to Dr. Erenberg), my mom and dad took me back to Cleveland for another appointment. Now that I am on medication, I have to see Dr. Erenberg regularly. At this appointment, Dr. Erenberg told my parents to increase my Chlondine to three quarters of a pill three times a day instead of only a half of a pill. He increased the dose to help with my behavior a little bit more. I asked Dr. Erenberg to help me with my hair pulling because my bald spots were being made fun of at school. Dr. Erenberg then told my parents and me about another drug called Zoloft that has been known to help with obsessive compulsive behaviors. My parents weren't too sure about another medicine so we decided to wait until the next visit to discuss it again.

In November I asked my parents to please let me try this new medicine because I couldn't stand pulling out my hair any more. They called Dr. Erenberg and ordered the medicine for me. I had to take one half of a pill once a day for a week. I added one half of a pill for three more weeks until I was taking two whole tablets once a day. My parents again had to call Dr. Erenberg to let him know how I was doing and if the medicine had any side effects. Zoloft, as far as I can tell, doesn't have any side effects. Zoloft seems to be working out great for me. I could tell from the first day that it was helping my Tourette because I came home from school happy. I'm never, ever happy after school because I'm under a lot of stress there. I'm also not happy after school because I know that I have home-work to do. I was still pulling out my hair and doing my facial tics, but not as often as I did before taking the Zoloft. I was also a whole lot nicer to my family and they were thrilled with me.

In early 1995, my parents, my brother and I went to the Cleveland Clinic for another appointment. My brother, Nicholas, wanted to go with us because we get to stay in a hotel with a swimming pool and he didn't want to miss out on the fun. He was also just curious about the Cleveland Clinic and Dr. Erenberg. At this visit Dr. Erenberg gave me a new medicine called "Orap." Orap is supposed to help with tics and it also can help make my Zoloft work better.

My head was almost bald on the top and Dr. Erenberg felt that this new medicine would help. At this visit, Dr. Erenberg said that it was O.K. to take me off my Chlondine for a while because my mom and dad didn't want me to take three different medicines at the same time. This was a very big mistake as I was miserable again.

I was sassing, saying bad words and I couldn't sit still. My mom, dad and I decided that it was best that I go back on the Chlondine, but with a smaller dose. Orap helped really well on my tics, but it makes me extremely tired and I gained a lot of weight.

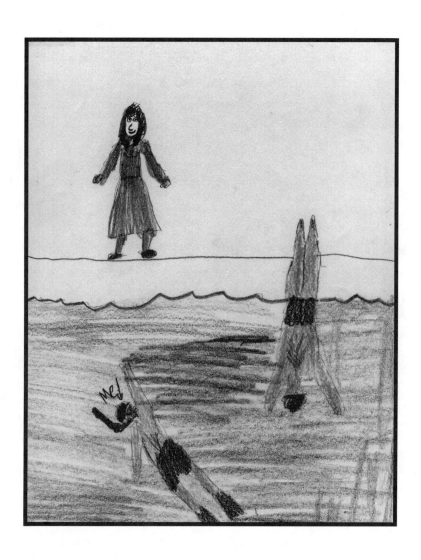

In August of 1995, my mom and I went
to the Cleveland Clinic with two friends that
have Tourette and their moms. We scheduled
our appointments together so that we could
share the ride to Cleveland. It also made the
time go faster because I had friends to talk to.
The only changes that Dr. Erenberg made on
this visit was increasing my Zoloft and
Chlondine and decreasing my Orap. This
change feels right because I'm not as tired and
I have lost some of the weight that I gained
before.

The second part of my treatment was
going to see Dr. Linda Ronald. She is a wonderful psychologist. When I was first diagnosed with Tourette, I was afraid of letting
people know because I thought they would
make fun of me.

Dr. Ronald helped make me more confi-
dent in telling my friends and classmates
about my problem. Dr. Ronald came to my
school and helped me show a Tourette video
to my class and then answered their questions
afterwards. The class' questions were really
good. One girl asked what it was like to have

Tourette. I answered by saying that Tourette has its advantages and its disadvantages. One advantage is that I really get into things and I don't want to give up. One disadvantage is that I have a lot of bald spots. Another question was asked on how I got Tourette. Dr. Ronald answered and said it was genetic and Igot it from my parents. A boy in my class asked how it felt to be teased about my problem. I told him that it hurt my feelings and that God made me special and I'm perfect just the way I am. One girl asked Dr. Ronald if my Tourette would go away. Dr. Ronald answered and told her that it would never go away. She also said that it could get better or it could get worse. There were other good questions, but I can't remember all of them. I was really excited and nervous about showing the video. Thinking about it made me shudder, but just knowing that Dr. Ronald was there to be my friend made it easier on me.

I had fun at Dr. Ronald's office. I haven't been to her office since the end of the fifth grade because my tics weren't causing me trouble and school was going pretty well. I can go back whenever I need to, but for now I am doing great. At Dr. Ronald's office, we had play sessions where we would play games. Some of the games helped me deal with stress, some were learning games and some were word games. We also painted pictures.

One visit I created a sandbox world with army men and dinosaurs and on other visits we played with puppets. One time my whole family came in and we performed a family puppet show. I had a great time doing that. Another fun visit was when Dr. Ronald filmed me telling my Tourette story. We made this film because some of the older kids in my school who don't know about my problem were making fun of me calling me "baldie." The film that I made was added to a movie that the Mental Health Association in town has on Tourette syndrome.

The Mental Health Association and Dr. Ronald came to my school and showed the film to all of the upper grades so that they could learn about my problem and stop teasing me. Dr. Ronald also did a demonstration on how it feels to have a tic. She made five students raise their right hand every time she slammed the desk with the video tape. They were supposed to write notes on material that was read to them. This was very hard for the students because their hands were constantly in the air and they didn't have very good notes to read when the demonstration was over. I'm really proud of Dr. Ronald for doing this to help me.

Aside from being a lot of fun, Dr. Ronald was also very helpful where school was concerned. Dr. Ronald went to school and talked with the principal and my teacher and explained my problem. She also explained what type of help I needed to be happy in school. Thanks to Dr. Ronald I now get to take my exams orally and I have less homework to do. Dr. Ronald tested my I.Q. during a visit and she said that I have "superior intelligence." That's why she felt that less homework wouldn't be harmful to me.

Dr. Ronald also recommended that I have an I.E.P. (Individual Educational Plan) to help me get through the sixth grade without frustration. The sixth grade is when middle school starts at my school. I change classes and have a lot more stress. The I.E.P. was written at the end of the fifth grade. My

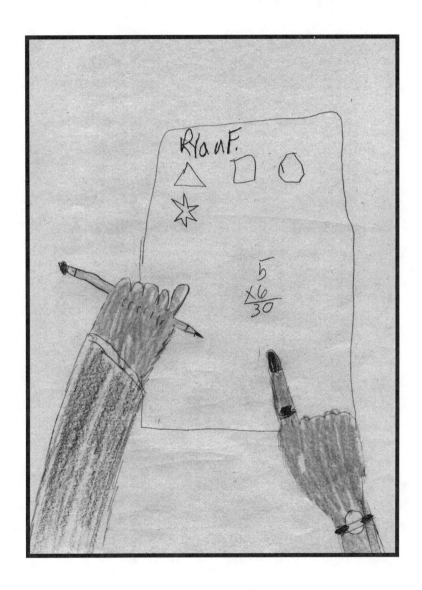

principal, Mrs. Hollingsworth (my fifth grade teacher), Dr. Ronald, the community school psychologist, a few of my sixth grade teachers and my parents all met at the end of the fifth grade to set up this plan.

The third part of my treatment is support from my family and my friends. My mom arranged for me to meet another child in town with Tourette syndrome. His name is Joseph.

Joseph has different Tourette symptoms than I do. When we first met, Joseph and I were both nervous. That didn't last long. That same night I had dinner over at his house and we found out that we were into the same things. Joseph collected "HeMan" figures like I did. Meeting Joseph was so helpful to me because it was great knowing that someone else in town had Tourette. Joseph has an older brother with Tourette. His name is Michael. Michael is a very talented artist. He created a sculpture of my brother and me called "Dedication" because I dedicated this book to my brother Nicholas and Nicholas is very dedicated to me. Joe and I meet regularly. We always have a great time and I really enjoy being around him. I have also met Lea and

Samantha at a support group for kids with T.S. at the park in town. I had a lot of fun that day because we played together and talked about our Tourette syndrome. This was easy because I knew that I was not being judged by these kids.

My family gives me a great deal of support. They pay a lot of money for my medicine, my therapy and my Cleveland visits. My parents never complain about the money, but it bothers me that they have to spend so much on me. My parents also support me in school by helping with my homework. When I was first diagnosed, my mom even asked our local hospital to put on a seminar on Tourette for the public. The hospital, on January 4, 1995, did this for us.

In April, 1995, my mom helped the Mental Health Association and our hospital put on an even larger workshop for the public. An Indianapolis neurologist was the featured speaker and there was a panel of five experts that also talked. I was asked to be a panelist for this workshop. I talked in front of doctors and nurses, parents, teachers, and friends. My speech covered my Tourette symptoms, my school, my teacher, my family and well, basically, my life. There was an article in the newspaper about me and the workshop. I was proud to be in this workshop because it was helpful to the community and it allowed me to prove to my teacher what I was capable of. My mom feels that workshops are very important for Tourette patients and their families. Educating the public on Tourette will stop the teasing.

My parents have also been a huge help in writing this book. I'm very grateful for all that they do.

••••••••••••••••••••••••

chapter five

The Fifth Grade

The first day of school was like every other first day of school, stressful. I was really scared. I was scared from the last day of fourth grade and every day during the summer about the first day of fifth grade. This time the first day was different because I was afraid of being teased about my Tourette. I didn't want anyone to know about my problem and I thought that I could hide it. Because of the facial tics and my many bald spots, I now know that I was wrong to think that I could hide it. Once I got to school, I felt a little more reassured because I knew I had a great teacher. She gave each student in the class a pencil that said "welcome back" on it.

My teacher's name was Mrs. Hollingsworth. She read all of the information that my parents had given her on Tourette syndrome over the summer and she knew a little bit about what it was going to be like having me in her classroom. I knew she had to be a great teacher because she went out of her way to learn about my problem before she ever met me. When Dr. Ronald (my therapist), the principal, my parents and Mrs. Hollingsworth all met at the beginning of the year, my teacher was given information by Dr. Ronald on how to help me enjoy my time at school. Some of the suggestions Dr. Ronald made were oral exams to make me less stressed and help me not pull out so many hairs. Another suggestion was to let me leave the classroom whenever I had to do my tics. I left the classroom a lot at the beginning of the year because I was embarrassed for anyone to see me doing my tics or pulling my hair out. No one understood that I couldn't stop pulling out my hair, so it was just as well that I left the room so that they couldn't see. I also left because I was afraid of being scolded for something that I couldn't control.

Another good suggestion that Dr. Ronald made was to limit the amount of homework that I have each night. If I had too much homework to do, I got stressed and pulled out my hair and did my tics. My behavior was bad

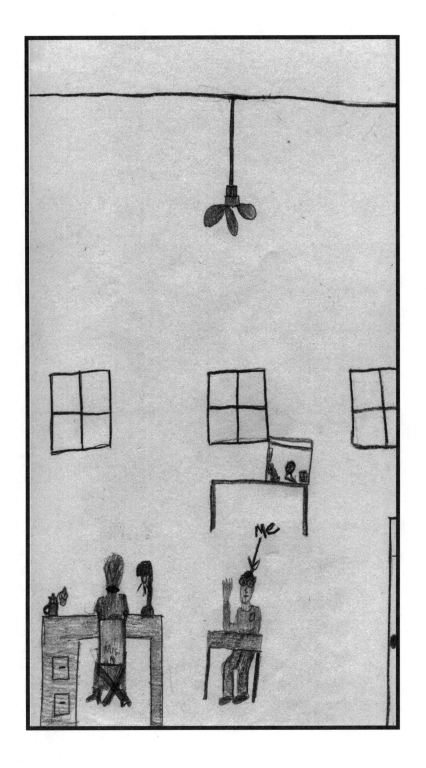

when I was stressed too. That's when I got mad at my parents and I ended up in trouble.

Mrs. Hollingsworth was very kind and helpful with Dr. Ronald's suggestions. With her help, I felt secure and was not afraid of going to school.

Sometimes I know I made Mrs. Hollingsworth really mad at me. I told you earlier that sometimes things just come out of my mouth and I can't stop them. I would blurt out inappropriate things at times when Mrs. Hollingsworth was teaching the class. I couldn't help myself. I know I hurt Mrs. Hollingsworth's feelings when I did this, but I would never do that on purpose. Mrs. Hollingsworth had such a tender heart and that's what I really loved about her.

Mrs. Hollingsworth encouraged me to keep trying my best. She rewarded me with "half homework assignments" when I controlled my talking out in class for three days at a time. She also gave me pencils, erasers and special stickers with the squirrels on them because she knew how obsessed I was with squirrel hunting. She allowed me to sit near her to keep me from being distracted. My ADHD made it hard for me to concentrate, and sitting right by her kept me focused on what I needed to be doing. Mrs. Hollingsworth allowed me to doze off in class at times. My medicine made me very sleepy and I fell asleep for a short time. Mrs. Hollingsworth was very understanding when this happened. I fell asleep off and on for about a week in school. Mrs. Hollingsworth also nominated me for a "Super Star Award" for trying my best. The principal selected the weekly "Super Star" from the names nominated by each teacher. I was selected the week before Christmas break. That's pretty amazing for me because I'm always extra excited and fidgety right before a holiday.

The principal, Mrs. Schlicte, helps encourage me in school also. She made it possible for me to wear my baseball cap in the building. Our dress code doesn't allow hats to be worn in school. Not all of the teachers knew at first that I had special permission to wear my hat inside. When they saw me wearing my hat, they told me to take it off. I was very upset and embarrassed when this happened. I would take off my hat when they

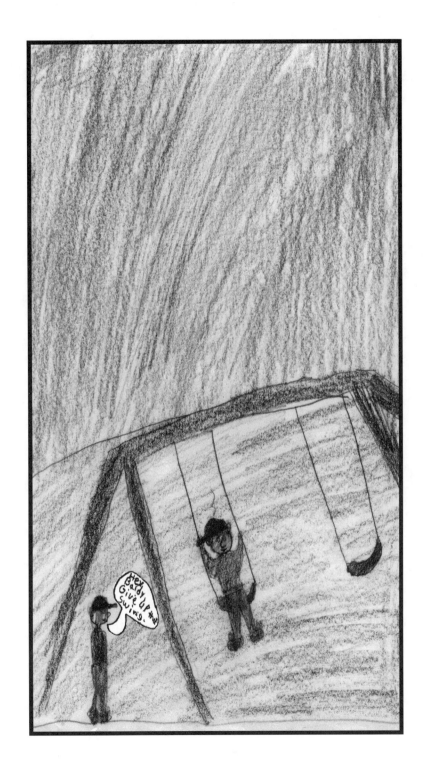

told me to because I didn't want to get in trouble for arguing with an adult. I now get to carry a laminated pass with me when I'm in school. It says that I have special permission to wear my hat in the building. The reason why my cap is so important to me is that it hides my bald spots and keeps the kids that do not know about my Tourette from making fun of me.

The office workers also support me. They give me my medication every day. I know they have a lot of work to do and I really appreciate them taking time out for me.

Not everyone in my school supported me. A lot of the kids were mean and cruel to me because of my Tourette. At the beginning of the year, some of the older kids in the sixth, seventh and eighth grades called me "baldie" and said very hurtful things to me. One person said, "It looks like you have Leukemia with those bald spots." Another person said, "You're getting old early because you're losing your hair." One boy said, "Your parents must be too poor to get you a hair cut, so they let your brother shave your head." One boy called me a "lizard" because of my facial tic. I've learned not to be bothered by the mean things that kids say to me because I know that there is nothing wrong with what I do. I have no control over what I do. The mean things that the older kids say aren't happening as often as they used to, but they are still happening. My parents say that these kind of kids are ignorant and need to be educated. This book should help do that.

Not all of the kids made fun of me. Some defended me when others made fun of me. Most of the fourth and fifth graders were nice to me. The kids in my class watched the Tourette video called "Stop It I Can't" early in the school year. Once they watched the video, they began apologizing for making fun of me in the past. They also were more understanding of the different things that my Tourette caused me to do and didn't hold them against me.

• •

chapter six

Summer Lessons

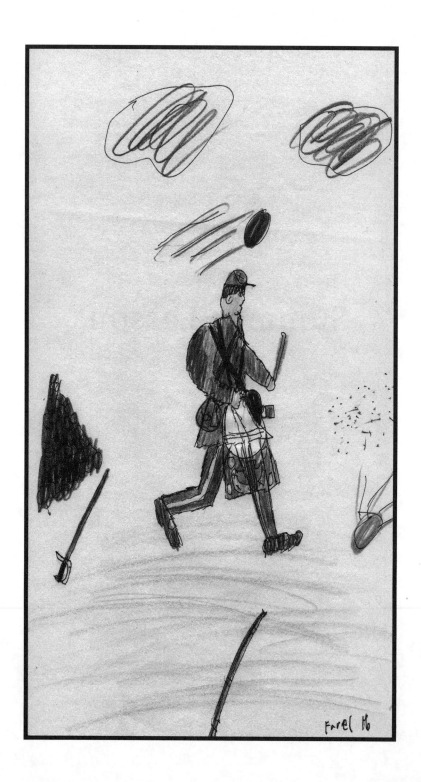

Summer was finally here! Once again there was no pressure from school. I was taking golf lessons, practicing to be a drummer boy, going to math tutoring with Mrs. Hollingsworth and just relaxing. My hair follicles even started to grow back. I was pretty happy. Things were going very well until something bad happened to me. I'd like to tell you about it.

On June 27, 1995, I invited my friend Jake over to spend the night. We slept out in my fort that my dad, my brother and I made. We were reenacting the Civil War in our back yard. All of the sudden, I heard my name being called from a fifteen-year-old neighbor boy. I thought he wanted to play Civil War with Jake and I, so we went over to see what he wanted. This boy was playing around with a BB gun in front of two other younger boys. I asked him if he wanted to play. He told me that his gun wasn't a fake. He then cocked the gun six times and loaded a BB into the chamber. This neighbor told me to run or he would shoot me. When I didn't run (because I thought he was kidding), he shot the BB gun. The BB went through my lip and shattered a permanent tooth on the lower left side of my mouth. I ran home and my mom rushed me to the oral surgeon's office. I was in intense pain and I thought that I was going to die. I had surgery to remove my tooth's root because the tooth had been completely shot out. Three days later, I had another surgery at the oral surgeon's office to remove the BB that had lodged in my jaw. My regular dentist found the BB lodged in my jaw when he was taking X-rays.

I'll bet you are wondering what happened to the boy that shot me. He came over to my house that same night I got shot. I was lying on the couch because I wasn't feeling too well. My mom asked me if I wanted to say anything to this boy. She wanted me to be able to get any anger out so I wouldn't have to carry it around with me. I told the boy that I forgave him and that I wanted to shake hands and be friends. My parents had the police destroy the gun and we didn't press charges. I know that God made me special because I was able to forgive him so quickly. One thing that my Tourette has taught me is how to forgive. I am so used to forgiving people for making fun of me.

A nicer lesson that I learned that summer was with the Boy Scouts. I went on my first real Boy Scout camping trip. I was a little upset because I had to leave my family. I was also excited at the same time because I got to camp in a tent with my buddy Jake and I earned six merit badges that week. The badges were tough to earn and I really worked hard on them. I learned about CPR, first aid, basketry, leather working, swimming, architecture and computers. I also learned to take care of myself without my Mom and Dad, made new friends and most importantly, I learned about responsibility. We had to keep our campsites clean, and our troop won an award for having the cleanest campsite. I wasn't made fun of once for my Tourette at camp. Boy, did that feel good!

On August 4, 1995 I learned that you can be famous and have Tourette. That day

I met Jim Eisenreich in Cincinnati at a Red's game. Jim Eisenreich plays left field for the Philadelphia Phillies. I felt like a king when I met him because he is so incredibly famous and he has Tourette like me. What a great guy he is!

•••••••••••••••••••••••••

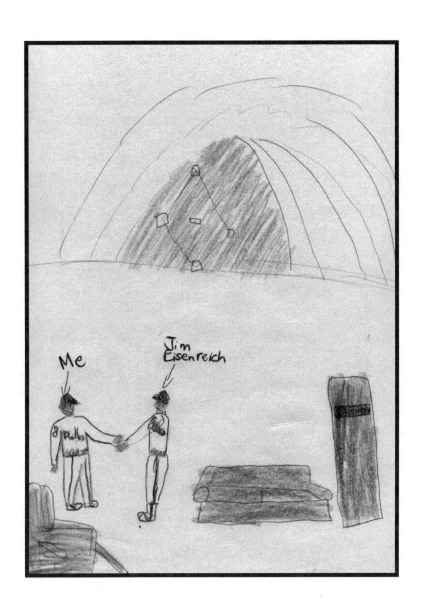

chapter seven

The Sixth Grade

The sixth grade is a lot different from the fifth grade. I have a lot more responsibilities than I did last year. I have more to remember and I have four teachers instead of only one like last year.

My homeroom teacher is Mr. Brown. He does so much to help me by reducing my stress. He meets weekly with my Mom to discuss any concerns about school. Before the meetings he talks with my other teachers about any problems that may be taking place in their classrooms. Mr. Brown always allows me to talk first at these weekly meetings. This feels good because I feel like I am being respected. Mr. Brown also teaches my science class. He believes in hands-on assignments rather than written assignments. This is a great stress reducer. Mr. Brown is also very fair and supportive. I'm very glad I'm in his class.

Miss Pace is my math teacher. She gives me reduced work because my I.E.P. recommends this. She is very nice to me and she makes me feel like I fit in. Math is a subject that I look forward to every day because of Miss Pace, and it is also the subject that stresses me out the most because of the concentration needed for it. I pull out my hair all of the time in math. It hurts, but it helps get rid of the mental distractions that are always going on in my head. Miss Pace also teaches my art class. She is the best artist I've ever seen. The projects are fun and interesting. Art is a real relaxing class.

Mrs. Young is my English, spelling and literature teacher. There is a lot of writing involved in these classes. I pull out my hair in these classes, too. Mrs. Young is also very nice and makes me feel good about myself.

Mrs. Culley is my religion teacher. She is the best religion teacher I've ever had. She is so full of love and kindness that she loves everybody. She also has a really cool dog named Alex who she brought to class one day. I've learned a lot about my religion this year because she calls on me all of the time. I like being called on because I'm not being ignored. I also stay focused this way.

Mr. Prybylla is my history, health and physical education teacher. I do not like history because we are learning world history. I only like U.S. history because of my Civil War obsession. I guess I also like U.S. history because of the American Revolution. I don't really care for health either. The only topic that is interesting in health is the skin. I liked the skin chapter because it covered hair and their follicles. I guess I don't need to remind you why I like those.

Physical education is fun because I get to run around and release energy. Releasing energy is real important for my ADHD. I'm able to sit still longer after I've been allowed to run around. Mr. Prybylla is a great gym teacher because he is a sporty kind of guy. He is also very helpful in history and health.

Another thing that is different about sixth grade is that I have cubicles in each of my classrooms that my parents donated to the school. I can work in them if I want to or I can just go in them to do my tics and pull out my hair. People can't see me pulling out my hair and that just makes me feel better.

I also get to take an extra set of my school books home to stay. This is because of my ADHD. Last year if I forgot my book for homework, I missed an assignment that I would have to make up later. Now if I forget a book it's not a big deal because I have one at home.

I have a lot of new friends this year. It gives me someone to talk to when I'm stressed about school and it also is more fun at recess time. One of my new friends, Jessica, is my math study buddy. She helps me when I struggle in math class. I'm a lot less stressed in math because of her.

My tests are still taken orally, but this year Mrs. Lewis is my testing aide. She writes the answers down for me which reduces my stress by a ton. It's still a test, but not half as hard as it would be if I had to do the writing.

Sixth grade is not as bad as I thought it was going to be. I have a lot of help and guidance by caring people and I'm very loved.

. . . .

chapter eight

My Family's Turn

My name is Karen, I'm Ryan's mother. Ryan and I decided that it would be both beneficial and important for his family to have a part in explaining Ryan's unique problem. Before I delve into Ryan's story, I feel it necessary to say something to you. Any of the feelings and stories I am about to put into the text of this book are in no way, shape or form meant to belittle or embarrass my son. It is only with the greatest amount of respect, admiration and unconditional love that I am able to write my thoughts down for his book.

Having said that, I'd like to tell you about the extra special gift I was given twelve years ago. I'm no different than any other mother when I say that my son was absolutely adorable. Ryan was a fun baby. He was so curious and happy and entertaining. I must say that he was exceptionally bright as well.

At the age of six months old he was capable of recognizing and pointing to items in a children's book that I would read to him. He also, at the age of six months, understood simple commands. Before leaving his room after a diaper change, I would ask him to turn off the light. He turned off the light. This simple task didn't surprise me until I was around other six-month-old children who weren't performing this type of function. He said simple words at seven months of age and would put two words together to form a simple question by nine months. His first question was "What's that?" Anyone who knows my curious son understands how humorous this question is. Ryan has the strongest need to know everything about everything that I have ever witnessed.

I would say that about the time Ryan was nine months old, his father and I knew that we were going to have our hands full. He started climbing out of his crib by using his stuffed animals as steps. He would throw his little leg over the bed rail and fall to the floor in a great thud! He didn't cry, he just chuckled to himself. I think he was both shocked and proud all at the same time. He would then crawl to us and say "Hi!" My husband and I were stunned. Nothing could keep Ryan from what Ryan wanted to do, not even the security of a crib. That's pretty much the way Ryan is now. He's a very determined, spirited young man. His Tourette just amplifies his determination and spirit.

Ryan's father, Steve, and I then began noticing some quirky behaviors in Ryan. At about nine months old, Ryan seemed to be set in his ways. I know it sounds funny, but he was. He had a system of going to bed. He had to kiss everything on the walls in his room before he would let us place him in his crib. If we went out of order with the kissing, Ryan would let us know by pointing to and telling us the objects. He would then direct us to the beginning and we would have to start all over. He began adding rooms of things to kiss and before we knew it, we were kissing the entire house good night. If we did not complete this nightly ritual, Ryan would not, under any circumstances, stop screaming until he got exactly what he wanted. We were beginning to wonder who was putting whom to bed!

Another quirk Ryan had, (Ryan mentioned this earlier) was smelling everything. Before he ate something, he had to smell it. When he opened a new toy or book, he had to give it a sniff. We thought this was so cute. We assumed that was his special way of exploring and quite honestly didn't think a thing of it. He still smells things; it is part of his Tourette.

Another "cute" habit that Ryan had was repeating things that people would say. For instance, one time I told Ryan not to touch something because he could get hurt. He instantly, like a tape recorder, repeated exactly what I had just said. Ryan did this all of the time. Again, we didn't think a thing of this either. It simply was Ryan's method of understanding what was said to him. Only occasionally will Ryan repeat things out loud now that he is older. Its amazing to watch his face when he repeats or does his echolalia. He's much like a computer processing data. You can clearly see his thought process at work.

We began noticing that, at around eighteen months of age, Ryan was obsessed with certain toys, things and people. Ryan had a blankie named "Patches" that his Grandma Farrell made when he was born. It went everywhere with us. So did his "funka." "Funka" was his favorite toilet plunger and it got its name from the sound it made. Shortly after this funka fascination started, we learned that I was expecting Ryan's little brother. Imagine the stares I was subjected to being a pregnant mother, toting a child, his blankie and his "funka"! Ryan would throw terrible temper tantrums if he was not allowed to carry these items in public. My mother (Grandma Coffee) bought Ryan a smaller funka to take out publicly. She felt that a smaller plunger would draw less stares. Ryan loved this little funka because his grandmother had given it to him, but the big funka still went out in public and that was the end of the subject as far as Ryan was concerned.

Ryan also was obsessed with certain people such as Tom Selleck, who starred on Magnum, P.I. (Ryan's favorite television program). Ryan constantly asked if his Thomas Magnum shorts were clean. I never noticed, but Magnum usually donned a pair of white shorts on the show. Ryan had to wear his white shorts after watching the show, and you can imagine what his response would be if his Magnum shorts were in the wash. Let's just say he became very aggravated. Through the years, Ryan has dressed up as many other characters as well as the important male figures in his life. The most recent is Lee Trevino, as Ryan is totally obsessed with golfing. Ryan's obsessive compulsive behaviors require him to be in some kind of "uniform" in order for him to feel adequate. I mentioned above that Ryan dressed up as Lee Trevino for a school book report. He not only dressed like Lee Trevino, but he carried in his golf bag and clubs as well. He couldn't think of being a famous golfer without first having the proper equipment with him. His obsession with accuracy earned him an "A" on the report.

There are so many stories like the few examples I just wrote that it would take another book just to share them. Suffice it to say that Ryan is very methodical and has to have things a certain way or else he becomes completely out of hand.

When Ryan's brother, Nicholas, was born, Ryan's systematic world had to be shared. Ryan's grandparents had to be shared,

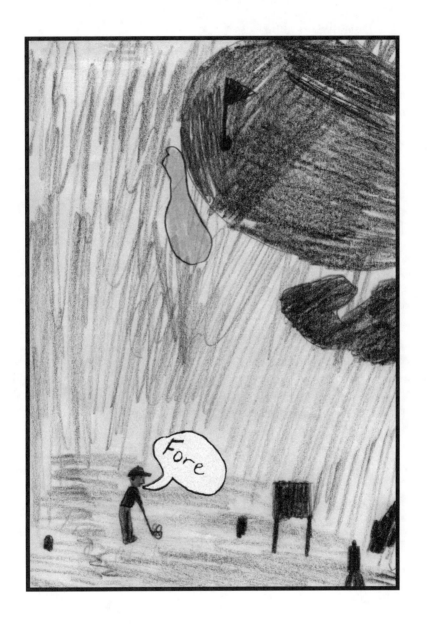

his parent's attention had to be shared, and worse yet, his toys had to be shared. This was extremely difficult for Ryan to handle. His behavior worsened. The fits were much more frequent and he became very controlling.

Ryan was almost two and one-half years old when Nicholas was born. Shortly thereafter, Ryan began playing with the "HeMan" figures. The characters usually carried some type of weapon. Ryan really poured himself into these toys. His every waking moment was spent on talking about or playing with these toys. The obsession with "HeMan" quickly turned into an obsession with weapons (mostly guns, swords and knives). Ryan mentioned in an earlier chapter that he slept with a sword down the back of his pajamas at night. He did this for at least two years.

Naturally, as parents, we were concerned about Ryan's fascination with weapons. Out of this concern, we took Ryan to a pediatric psychologist at the age of three and one-half. The doctor felt there was no reason to be alarmed by Ryan's behaviors given the fact that my three brothers were policemen and that Ryan's father was a hunter.

Ryan was just very imaginative. That's what we wanted to hear, but we still felt that Ryan's behaviors weren't quite normal.

Once Kindergarten started at age five, Ryan's story becomes even more complex. We noticed that Ryan's unique spirit, the one that we thought was so cute, was causing him considerable difficulty. He was outspoken, he fibbed frequently and with great skill, I might add, and he was having difficulty following directions. My husband and I began noticing that Ryan's behavior worsened and his concentration level fell during periods of anxiety. By anxiety, I mean good or bad stress. Ryan could not deal with unexpected events like quizzes in school. He also had a hard time dealing with the anticipation of holidays and his birthday. You could almost mark your calendar a month to the day before a holiday, vacation or birthday by Ryan's behavior. He would lose all concentration and become totally uninhibited about what came out of his mouth. The teachers, year after year, convinced us that Ryan was just all boy. Again, that's what we wanted to hear, but we still knew there was more to Ryan than being all boy. We played along with the "all boy" story up until the third grade.

Halfway through the third grade, we felt compelled to have Ryan tested for ADHD. We didn't know much about ADHD, but from what we had been told about the disorder, Ryan certainly was exhibiting all of the behaviors necessary to diagnose him with it. We were totally unaware of the social worker's lack of discretion when she pulled Ryan from class to be tested. We heard that story for the first time when Ryan wrote it in this book. We were totally amazed that someone who constantly interacts with children could have so little respect for them. As Ryan indicated, he was diagnosed with ADHD. Finally, we had an answer or so we thought.

As a family, we went into counseling to learn the proper behavior management tactics. They were remarkably effective for about a year and a half. Ryan repeated the third grade after a lot of soul searching on my husband's and my part. We felt that given Ryan's diagnosis of ADHD, and his immaturity, we owed him a year to get caught up. We explained to Ryan that we made a mistake and had pushed him too hard by starting him in school at such a young age. Ryan went along with our conclusion and I'm certain he felt somewhat relieved by it.

Ryan seemed once again to be our curious, happy, entertaining little boy. Things went pretty well the year Ryan repeated third grade and actually through half of the fourth grade year. Fourth grade, as you may recall, was in a new city. Ryan then became obstinate, rude, hateful and just plain miserable. Doing homework with Ryan was a complete nightmare. He wanted my help, but he wasn't willing to take it. He threw fits, threw pencils and became destructive. He would bring up past punishments that had no relevance to his homework and would sidetrack himself so much that neither of us knew which end was up. I truly felt despised on a daily basis. I knew that he hated himself for being this way as well. To make matters worse, Ryan began making these strange faces. He would widen his eyes, stretch his mouth as wide as it could and then stick out his tongue. This function was constant. When I tried asking him why he was doing this, he simply replied, "Doing what?" At around the same time as these new facial tics began happening, I noticed that Ryan had a bald spot on the back of his head. He was pulling out his own hair! I couldn't believe that Ryan would want to physically harm himself. To my astonishment, Ryan was completely unaware that he was pulling out his hair.

Ryan explained how we met Dr. Erenberg, so I won't go though the details again. I will add, however, that I was thoroughly impressed with Dr. Erenberg. He was extremely professional and caring. I realize that this incredible man sees hundreds of patients in a week, but I witnessed Dr. Erenberg making Ryan feel that he was the most important patient he had ever seen. June 2, 1994 was the most liberating day as a parent that I have ever known. We had a reason for Ryan's behavior. Our (my husband's and my) suspicions were confirmed. There was more to Ryan than ADHD and being "all boy"! Tourette syndrome. What a beautiful name. Our son wasn't purposefully doing all those bizarre things. They were attributed to something medical. The "pity parties" we had been having were over and we saw the light at the end of the tunnel! We began the process of helping our son cope with his rare problem.

I'd be lying to you and myself if I said that Ryan's Tourette has been easy on our family. We have had to make many concessions where Ryan is concerned and they haven't been without cost. Nicholas, our other incredibly special son, has many times unfairly assumed the role of being the oldest child simply to keep Ryan from exploding. Nicholas' self assumed role often led him to feel responsible for fixing Ryan's Tourette. Nick would lay out Ryan's medication for him so that he wouldn't forget, as Ryan without medication was not a pretty sight. Nick would also forego time with my husband and me to allow Ryan more than his share of attention. He also found himself taking on extra chores so that Ryan wouldn't have to get upset by having too much to do. We worked on rebuilding our family unit with the help of Dr. Ronald. It was a wonderful process.

Ryan's Tourette has been a blessing in many ways. Not only are we becoming a stronger family, but we are gaining considerable knowledge about Tourette. It's this

knowledge that we have gained that has
empowered us to lovingly cope with Ryan on
a daily basis. We're hoping that the empower-
ment we've attained can serve other families
in the same situation. I have helped our local
Mental Health Association provide a half day
workshop on Tourette syndrome in which
Ryan was an expert panelist. I must admit
that Ryan stole the show from our featured
speaker. I do not believe there was a dry eye
in the house after Ryan completed his oration.
He is becoming quite the public speaker as he
has been asked by several associations to
address the issues of Tourette. Ryan and I are
attempting to get the public educated and cre-
ate an awareness of the disorder.

Another blessing I've witnessed is Ryan's
total acceptance of his disorder. When Ryan
was first diagnosed with Tourette, he wanted
no one to know because he was fearful of
negative reactions. With the help of his med-
ications, caring medical professionals and
family support, Ryan has come full circle with
his emotions. He believes, as I do, that his
Tourette is a gift given to him for sharing with
others struggling with their own acceptance of
this fascinating disorder.

Life isn't a picnic for my son. I told you about Ryan's one bald spot earlier in the chapter. Since his diagnosis, his one spot has grown to many. If Ryan continues pulling out his hair at his present rate, he will become completely bald. Simple tasks such as reading frustrate Ryan because of the repetitive reading his Tourette forces him to execute. Going to church is very stressful for Ryan, as well. Most children Ryan's age have absolutely no trouble sitting through a one hour service. It's torture for Ryan. He begs me to either hold his hands so that he can't tug at his hair or to rub his head to help his "tingle" go away. He fidgets, taps, squirms, shifts and pulls his hair for the solid hour. You can't believe the stares we are subjected to by unknowing parishioners. One Sunday morning an older couple spotted Ryan with his cap on during service. These folks were unaware of Ryan's special circumstances and of the fact that Ryan has permission to wear his cap in church. They promptly asked him to remove it. Ryan, taking the matter into his own capable hands, tried to explain that he is allowed to wear his cap because of his balding head and his Tourette. They repeated their request to remove his hat even after Ryan's eloquent reasoning. People

who are quick to judge and who are unedu-
cated about Tourette can be quite maddening
if you allow it to consume you. My recom-
mendation to Ryan on how to deal with this
couple in church was to extend his hand in
friendship at the "sign of peace" portion of
mass. Ryan felt better and I'm sure this couple
was humbled by his simple gesture of peace.

If I can leave you with just an inkling of
what it must be like to be in this little guy's
mind, I'd be content. Ryan not only has to deal
with the everyday frustrations of growing up
and going to school, but he deals on a daily
basis with ridicule, embarrassment, and total
frustration. It's this same child who is writing
from his heart to try and help those suffering
with Tourette syndrome and to forgive those
who cause these sufferings. God did make
Ryan special, he just isn't aware of how
incredibly special he is!

••••••••••••••••••••••••

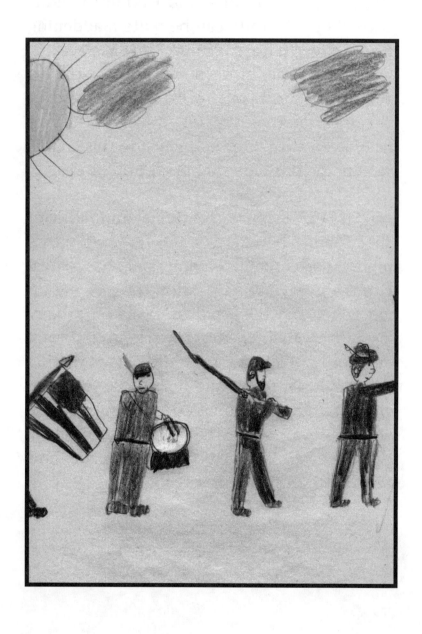

Hi, I'm Nick. I'm 10 years old, and I'm Ryan's brother. Sometimes I feel mad at my family because Ryan gets so much of the attention. I know my family loves me, but I still get mad at Ryan's Tourette because if he didn't have it, he wouldn't get the attention of our mom and dad. I also get mad at Ryan's Tourette because sometimes he isn't very nice to me. He says he's sorry when he's mean to me, and most of the time I forgive him. I love my brother, even though it's hard, so I put up with his Tourette.

I feel sad for Ryan when kids make fun of him on the bus. One time a kid made fun of the faces Ryan makes. I stood up for Ryan when that happened. I told him to leave Ryan alone because he can't help it. I also feel sad for my mom and dad when Ryan gets mad at them. When Ryan gets mad at his homework, he takes it out on my mom or on me. I'm sad for Ryan at the same time.

Most of the time Ryan is nice to me because he doesn't have very many friends. I play what he wants to play (which is mostly the Civil War) instead of what I want to play.

Sometimes that leaves me with no time to play what I want to play.

Sometimes I'm jealous of Ryan because he gets to wear his hat in school. I can understand why he needs his hat, but I'd like to wear one too! Ryan gets jealous of me too! I get good grades in school and never study, but Ryan struggles when he studies for tests. That makes us about even. I'm jealous of him and he is jealous of me.

I'm very proud of Ryan for writing this book. I know I couldn't do it. It will probably help other kids like Ryan feel good about themselves and it will let them know that they aren't the only ones with Tourette. I'm also very proud that Ryan dedicated this book to me. It made me warm inside and made me want to cry... and I did.

••••••••••••••••••••••••••

chapter nine

What's Ahead For Me?

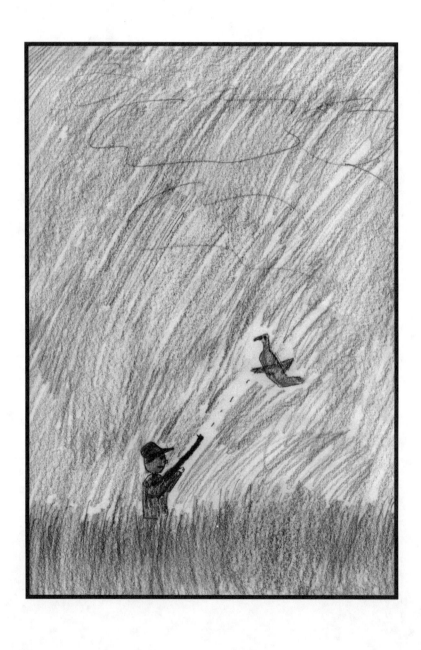

The future is very scary for me. I think that's true for anyone, whether they have Tourette syndrome or not. I'm afraid of not being accepted for who I am. I won't always attend the school I go to now and the thought of making new friends scares me. I've done that before and some of my friends have used my Tourette against me. I'm content with the friends that I have now.

I plan on attending college like a lot of other people. My interests are constantly changing, so I do not know what my major will be. Some of my interests now include hunting (this will always interest me), golfing and Tourette. I might try to become a neurologist like Dr. Erenberg. I really want to help Tourette patients whether I become a doctor or not. Whatever I choose for a career, I will try my best. My Obsessive Compulsive behavior helps me to stay focused on whatever I'm into at the time.

My Tourette has helped me to learn something about my hobbies and sports activities. I only like individual sports, not team sports. Team sports make me stressed. I have been on basketball, soccer and baseball teams before. Each team made me miserable because I wasn't a great player. Some of the kids would make fun of me and make me nervous. This made me do my tics nonstop. I now get to choose which sports I participate in. I like archery, target shooting, golfing and hunting. I am also involved with Scouting. I like the Scouts because the activities are interesting to me. I do not get stressed in Scouts and the kids treat me with respect.

I plan on getting married and having a family some day. When I first got the diagnosis for Tourette, I told my Mom that I didn't want to have a family because I didn't want my children to have Tourette like me. Now that I know that having Tourette is O.K., I'm not as worried about that.

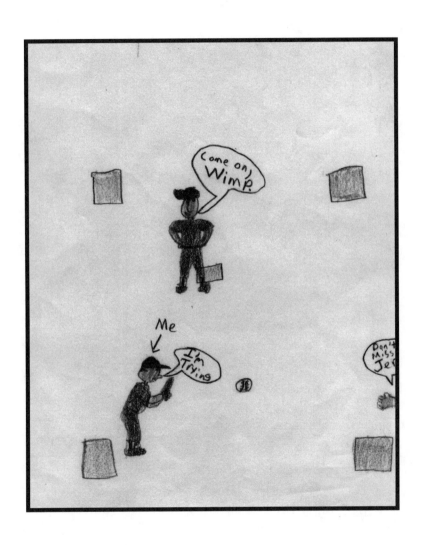

I think I'm lucky that God made me special because I know that I will be a success in life. Tourette has taught me to be a good friend, a good son and a good person. Anything that does all of this can't be all bad. For those of you who have Tourette, find out what you want to do and go for it! Don't use your Tourette as an excuse to stop you from getting what you want. For those of you who do not have Tourette syndrome, hopefully this book will make you stop and think before you tease someone who does. They can't help themselves and they don't need a reminder that they are different. They are perfect just the way they are.

....

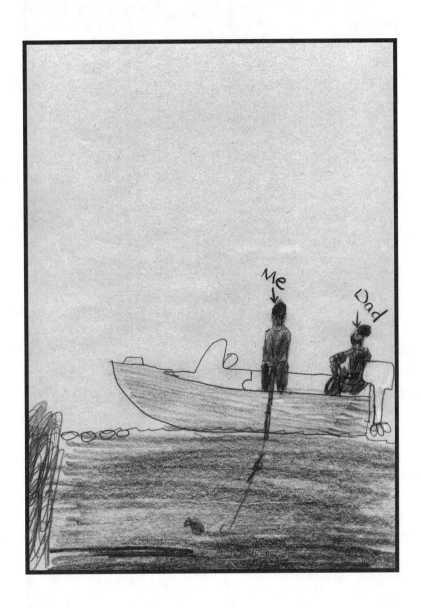

BIBLIOGRAPHY

This brief Bibliography is included to give the reader a place to start. It is by no means inclusive or complete. Please take the time to visit your local library or call any Tourette Syndrome Association in your area or the National Tourette Syndrome Association at 718. 224. 2999 for more information.

TOURETTE SYNDROME

Children With Tourette Syndrome. Haerle, Tracy (1992)

Living With Tourette Syndrome. Shimberg, Elaine (1995)

Hi, I'm Adam. Buehrens, Adam (1991)

Ryan. Hughes, Susan (1996)

What Makes Ryan Tick. Hughes, Susan (1996)

Tourette Syndrome and Human Behavior. Comings, David, M.D.

GENERAL

It's Nobody's Fault. Koplewicz, Harold, M.D. (1996)

Parenting A Child With ADHA. Boyles, Nancy M.Ed., Contdino, Darlene, Ph.D. (1995)

Lonely, Sad and Angry. Ingersoll, Barbara, Ph.D., Pruitt, Sheryl, M.Ed. (1995)

What "Ronald" Would Like You To Know
About His Foundation

Ronald McDonald House Charities (RMHC) is a not-for-profit organization that "lifts kids to a better tomorrow" by supporting the Columbus Ronald McDonald House—a home-away-from-home for the families of seriously ill children in Columbus area hospitals—and providing grants to community organizations aimed at helping children and families of Central Ohio.

The Columbus House was established in 1982 and has 30 bedrooms, 2 kitchens, 12 bathrooms, 2 laundry rooms, a playroom, and several common areas for our families to use. The House serves approximately 1,200 families from the Central Ohio area every year.

In addition to RMHC's continued commitment to the Columbus Ronald McDonald House, RMHC has awarded Awards and Grants to local children's charities in a 21-county area. RMHC funds projects in the areas of health care and medical research, social and civic concerns, and education.

NOTES